Top 50 Best "Stress Busting" Smoothies

Stress Management Made Easy

Treat yourself to these easy nutritious creamy rich delicious "stress busting" smoothies at breakfast, or any time of day, and fill your body with loads of nutrients, including protein, vitamins, minerals, amino acids and enzymes, for stress relief, to build your resilience to stress, and to calm your frazzled nerves.

Stressful situations are often unavoidable, but something as simple as a smoothie a day, or even as needed, can make all the difference in the world to how well you hold up to stressful situations, and how well you rebound from stress, so your immune system doesn't become impaired by stress, and you don't find yourself sick as a result of being over stressed, seeking help from your practitioner, or worse, when some basic stress relief could have, and may still, work wonders.

Stress is the polar opposite of the deep relaxing, delta wave rest state needed for rejuvenation and a well-functioning immune system. A delicious healthy smoothie could easily complement anything else you might be doing, including coping with challenges and conditions like stress, anxiety and depression.

Become a Stress Buster Today, with "Stress Busting" Smoothies...

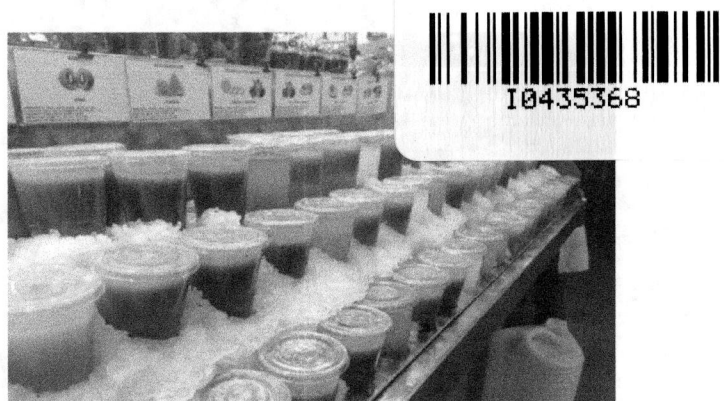

I0435368

As a Thank You for your interest in Dan Harp's books, he has included a few bonus sections for you, in addition to Smoothie Preparation and Top "Stress Busting" Smoothies.

Bonus 1 - Top "Stress Busting" Superfoods

Bonus 2 - Top "Stress Busting" Juices

Bonus 3 - Top "Stress Busting" Tips

Healthy Vibrations Contact Form Information:
http://www.highlyvibrantwellbeing.com/contact-us.html

Extra... Extra... Extra... Bonus 4... if you purchased any of Dan Harp's books, including this one, you are hereby authorized to distribute this book, in any format, as a gift to immediate family and close friends, without concern about copyright infringement, as long as it is distributed in its entirety, without changes, with the copyright notice intact.

Ordering Information:

Quantity sales - Special discounts are available on quantity purchases by corporations, associations, and others. For details, contact the publisher at the email address above.

This book is available at Amazon.com in Paperback, Kindle, and Any Device Editions. Some of Dan Harp's Other Books are available through the Kindle Unlimited Program.

This book is also available at iBookstore, Kobo, B&N Nook, Smashwords (ePub, Mobi, PDF, LRF, PDB, HTML, Text), Best Indie Book Store (ePub, Mobi, PDF) and various independent book stores.

All formats are available DRM-free, because we trust anyone who can enjoy a delicious smoothie and is interested in personal growth and a healthier lifestyle. Other books by Dan Harp, including paperback editions, can be found at Author Central.

Author Central
http://www.amazon.com/author/danharp

Smoothie Preparation...

For green smoothies, you can generally take your choice of beet root tops, collard greens, dandelion, kale, lettuce, parsley, spinach, and Swiss chard. The fruit usually does a good job of hiding the bitterness of the greens, but substitutions may take some experimenting.

The body metabolizes proteins quickly under stress, so replenishing them is essential to fully relieve stress. Some recipes include peanut butter, flaxseed or nuts. Another way to go is to add two scoops of natural protein powder to any smoothie, shake or juice to round things out.

Another ingredient you can add to any smoothie is a tablespoon Organic Superfood and/or Green Powder. These can also help relieve stress, increase energy, and boost mood.

For best results, use pre-sliced frozen bananas, apples, avocados, mangos and berries (frozen for at least two hours in the freezer), but in a rush, you can always throw in some ice cubes or cold water to top off these smoothies.

Whenever possible, use organic produce, especially with carrots, celery, cucumber, apples, berries and greens, otherwise, wash thoroughly with warm water and chop of at least one inch from the top of carrots.

Most smoothies can use your choice of milk or low-fat milk, but for stress relief, almond milk and coconut milk are your best choices.

Bonus 1 - Top "Stress Busting" Superfood Ingredients...

Bananas have potassium, which helps regulate blood pressure at times of stress, along with manganese and Vitamin B6, which helps produce serotonin, the happiness and feel good hormone.

Flaxseed is a powerhouse of nutrition, with Omega-3 essential oils which reduce stress, along with protein which helps to replenish depleted resources from stress. It offers so many benefits against cancer, diabetes, cholesterol, blood pressure, digestion, asthma, arthritis, and inflammation.

Mangos are known as the "King of Fruit", contains the linalool compound which has antidepressant and anti-anxiety effects, protects against cancer, diabetes and strokes, prevents early ageing and degenerative disease, improves eye health, lowers cholesterol and triglycerides, improves immunity, improves skin health, and improves digestion.

Blueberries have anthocyanins that increase production of dopamine in the brain, a chemical critical to coordination, memory function, and your mood.

Pineapples are rich in Vitamin C, Magnesium, and Serotonin, which helps reduce stress, improves digestion, accelerates healing, strengthens the immune system, increases protein availability by reducing dehydration, lowers blood cholesterols, helps fight cancer, helps with weight loss, sore throats, bloating, inflammatory skin, and dandruff.

Fruits high in antioxidants, Vitamin C and Magnesium, including oranges (citrus fruits), strawberries (berries), papaya, avocados, bananas, pineapples, mangoes, guavas, kiwifruit and tomatoes are recognized as stress reducing by lowering cortisol levels. Studies have shown that fruits and vegetables of any kind can help calm the nerves, feeling calmer, happier and more energetic.

Yogurt eases stress, anxiety and depression, by blocking emotion and pain and help keep a "feel good" state of mind. Probiotics can change the makeup of your gut flora making you more stress resilient.

Coconut Oil is often considered more effective than drugs at combating stress and depression. **Coconut water** contains minerals that help to rebalance electrolyte levels to help keep you calm.

Dark Chocolate provides a mood burst, increasing anandamide, a brain neurotransmitter that blocks pain, anxiety and depression, along with other chemicals that prolong the "feel-good" aspects of anandamide.

Peanut Butter makes you less likely to develop heart related issues or type-2 diabetes, despite the sugar and fat content, and it's a great source of protein which is necessary to replenish at times of stress.

Spinach is loaded with magnesium, which helps with general fatigue, along with folate, which helps your body produce mood-regulating neurotransmitters.

Kale is very high in vitamins, minerals and antioxidants that are effective for stress, liver function, prevention of cancer and Alzheimer's, is an effective anti-inflammatory, supports the cardiovascular system, vision, skin, immune system, and metabolism, and is a great detox food because of the high sulfur and fiber content.

Seeds, nuts, green leafy vegetables like spinach, seaweed, avocados and Swiss chad are all excellent sources of magnesium, which is well known for numerous benefits, including reduced anxiety, panic attacks, depression, fatigue, and headaches, improves sleep and helps regulate serotonin, energy, emotions, and wellbeing.

Vegetables that are particularly good for stress relief includes kale, spinach, seaweed, broccoli, beet, asparagus, cabbage, and cilantro.

Pomegranate lowers the stress hormone cortisone, improves memory, has impressive anti-inflammatory effects, helps lower blood pressure, helps fight cancer, arthritis and joint pain, bacterial infections and fungal infections, and lowers your risk of heart disease.

Avocados have about 20 essential health-boosting nutrients, helps curb appetite, helps regulate blood sugar levels, is a good source of magnesium, and helps to keep your mood steady, even at times of stress.

Ginger helps to boost your mood and clear out chemicals secreted by the body that leads to stress from being worried.

Vanilla bean helps calm, soothe, and relax the body and it's smell activates the feel-good sensations in the brain.

Cinnamon improves mood, alertness, memory, brain function and depression, helps control blood sugar levels, digestion, IBS – Irritable Bowel Syndrome, weight loss, cholesterol, triglycerides, and is an antioxidant, antibacterial, antimicrobial, and even helps fight stomach bugs, flu, cold, E-coli, sore throat, cough, salmonella, and candida yeast infections. It also helps prevent cancer, arthritis, osteoporosis, Alzheimer's disease, Parkinson's disease, and gum disease.

The Top "Stress Busting" Smoothies...

Nutty Banana Smoothie

Ingredients

- 1 tablespoon peanut butter
- 1 banana
- Hand full of berries
- 1 tablespoon raw honey
- Splash of almond milk

Blueberry Banana Almond Smoothie

Ingredients

- 1 cup blueberries
- 1 banana
- ½ cup almond milk

Orange Peach Mango Smoothie

Ingredients

- 2 oranges
- 1 cup diced peaches
- 1 cup diced mango
- A few ice cubes

The Orange Banana Carrot Smoothie

Ingredients – Two Servings

- 2 bananas
- 1 cup orange juice
- 1 orange
- 1 carrot
- ¾ cup almond milk
- 1 teaspoon vanilla extract

Dark Chocolate Walnut Banana Apple Green Smoothie

Ingredients

- 1 banana
- 1 apple
- 2 tablespoons cacao nibs
- ¼ cup walnuts
- 1 cup vanilla almond milk
- 1½ ounces baby spinach

Banana Orange Apple Berries Green Smoothie

Ingredients

- 1 bananas
- 1 orange
- 1 apple
- 1 cup mixed berries
- 1 tablespoon flaxseed
- 1 cup spinach
- 1 cup mango or pineapple tropical juice

Banana Berry Pineapple Carrot Green Smoothie

Ingredients

- 1 banana
- A handful of mixed berries
- A few slices of fresh pineapple
- One carrot
- ½ a celery stock
- A large handful of green leafy vegetables
- A few ice cubes

Avocado Mint Fennel Pineapple Smoothie

Ingredients

- 8 leaves of fresh mint
- 2 slices of avocado
- ½ cup fresh chopped fennel
- ½ can crushed pineapple in juice, not syrup

Banana Pineapple Coconut Smoothie

Ingredients

- 1 banana
- ½ can crushed pineapple in juice, not syrup
- ½ tablespoon coconut oil
- 1 tablespoon of shredded coconut

Banana Grapefruit Kale Honey Coconut Smoothie

Ingredients

- 1 banana
- A large handful of kale
- ½ pink grapefruit
- 1 tablespoon raw honey
- 1 tablespoon coconut oil

Banana Strawberry Green Smoothie

Ingredients

- 2 ripe bananas
- one large handful of fresh or frozen strawberries
- ½ head of romaine lettuce
- 2 cups cold water or ice cubes

Banana Mango Coconut Date Green Smoothie

Ingredients

- 2 bananas
- 1 cup ripe mango, chopped
- 1 cup young thai coconut water
- 3 pitted medjool dates
- ½ teaspoon vanilla bean powder
- 1 cup cucumber
- 3 celery stalks

Blueberry Coconut Green Smoothie

Ingredients

- 1-2 cups fresh or frozen blueberries
- 1-2 cups coconut
- 1-2 cups lettuce of choice
- ½ cucumber

Apple Avocado Green Smoothie

Ingredients

- 2 apples
- 1 avocado
- 1 handful of spinach
- 3 tablespoons chia seeds
- 1 cup of water

Pineapple Kiwi Cashews Green Smoothie

Ingredients

- 4 ounces pineapple
- 1 kiwi, peeled
- 1½ ounces baby kale
- ½ teaspoon matcha powder
- ¼ cup raw cashews
- 1 cup water

Banana Orange Lemon Chamomile Mint Green Smoothie

Ingredients

- 1 banana
- 1 orange
- ½ lemon
- 2 tablespoons chamomile flowers
- 1 ½ oz Swiss chard
- 1 tablespoons chia seeds
- 2 sprigs fresh mint
- 1 cup water

Avocado Almond Dates Green Smoothie

Ingredients

- ¼ ripe avocado
- ¾ cup unsweetened almond milk
- 1 tsp smooth unsalted almond butter
- 3 dates, pitted
- Handful of baby spinach
- 1 teaspoon vanilla extract
- 4-5 drops liquid Stevia, to taste (optional)
- 1 teaspoon whole chia seeds, to serve

Nectarine Orange Strawberry Coconut Vanilla Smoothie

Ingredients

- 5 nectarines
- 1 cup freshly squeezed orange juice
- 1 cup fresh or frozen strawberries
- 1 cup young thai coconut water (or regular water)
- ½ teaspoon vanilla bean powder

Blueberry Banana Coconut Flaxseed Cinnamon Smoothie

Ingredients

- 1 cup fresh or frozen blueberries
- 1 small ripe organic banana
- 1½ cups coconut water
- 2 teaspoons ground flaxseeds
- pinch of cinnamon
- ½ teaspoon vanilla extract

Apple Blueberry Avocado Ginger Smoothie

Ingredients

- 1 apple
- 1 handful blueberries
- ¼ Avocado
- 1 chunk ginger.
- 1 handful spinach
- 1 tablespoon chia seeds
- Top off with coconut water

Mango Coconut Orange Vanilla Smoothie

Ingredients

- 3 cups of mango or 3 small mangos
- 1 can of coconut milk
- 1 cup of orange juice or water
- 1 teaspoon of vanilla extract

Banana Peanut Butter Green Smoothie

Ingredients

- 1 bananas
- 2 tablespoon almond butter (can also use peanut butter)
- 1 tablespoon flax seed
- 4 large leaves or equivalent of smaller leaves of kale (take the rib out)
- 8 oz. or to taste of almond milk

Avocado Almond Green Shake

Ingredients

- ¼ ripe avocado
- ¾ cup almond milk
- 1 teaspoon smooth unsalted almond butter
- 3 dates, pitted
- handful of baby spinach
- 1 teaspoon vanilla extract
- 4-5 drops liquid Stevia, to taste (optional)
- 1 tsp whole chia seeds, to serve

Avocado Orange Blueberry Pineapple Green Smoothie

Ingredients

- 1 avocado
- ½ orange
- ½ cup blueberries
- ½ cup pineapple
- 2 tablespoons cashew butter
- 1 cup kale
- ¼ cup ice
- 1 teaspoon vanilla extract

Banana Pumpkin Flaxseed Green Smoothie

Ingredients

- 1 banana
- 2 smallish dates
- 2 big handfuls fresh spinach
- ¾ cup pumpkin puree
- 1 cup nut milk of your choice
- 1 tablespoon flax seed
- a few shakes of cinnamon
- a few shakes of pumpkin pie spice
- 8 ice cubes

Kiwi Strawberry Mango Mint Flaxseed Green Smoothie

Ingredients

- 1 small kiwi or half a large kiwi
- 5 fresh or frozen strawberries
- ½ of mango
- 1 tablespoon flax seed
- 3 cups of spinach
- handful of fresh mint
- squeeze of half a lemon
- ½ a frozen banana
- ½ cup of water

Banana Cinnamon Green Smoothie

Ingredients

- 1 frozen banana
- 1 cup almond milk
- ¾ cups kale leaves
- 1 tablespoon almond butter or other nut butter
- 1 tablespoon flax seed
- pinch of cinnamon, ginger and nutmeg
- 3-4 ice cubes

Pineapple Banana Apple Date Green Smoothie

Ingredients

- ¼ cup pineapple
- ½ banana
- 1 golden apple
- 2 cup frozen, chopped greens such as collards, kale, or spinach
- 1 tablespoon flax seed
- 1-2 medjool dates (de-seeded)
- 2 cups of water

Banana Apple Pineapple Yogurt Green Smoothie

Ingredients

- 1 banana
- ½ cup apple
- ½ cup pineapple
- 2 cups spinach
- yogurt
- 1 cup almond milk
- 1 tablespoon flax seed

Apple Green Smoothie

Ingredients

- 2 cups apples
- 2 handfuls greens
- 1 tablespoon flax seed
- 1 cup water

Banana Blueberry Almond Green Smoothie

Ingredients

- 1 banana
- ½ cup blueberries
- 1 cup almond milk
- 2 cups fresh spinach
- 1 tablespoon flax seed

Banana Vanilla Green Smoothie

Ingredients

- 1 banana
- organic spinach
- Swiss chard
- 1 cup vanilla almond milk

Green Smoothie

Ingredients

- kale
- chard
- carrot
- half a stalk of celery
- vanilla almond milk
- 3-4 dates
- dash of cinnamon
- 2 tablespoon hemp seeds
- 1 tablespoon flax seed
- chunk of cucumber
- ice

Berry Mango Carrot Lemon Grape Banana Green Smoothie

Ingredients

- 1 cup fresh or frozen mixed berries,
- 1 cup mango
- 2 carrots
- ½ lemon with skin
- ½ cup frozen black grapes
- ½ frozen banana
- 1 tablespoon green tea powder (matcha) or 2 tablespoons green tea
- 1 tablespoon whole flax seed
- 1 teaspoon bee pollen
- Handful of spinach
- 1 cup water

Banana Grapefruit Green Smoothie

Ingredients

- 1 banana
- ½ pink grapefruit
- 2 big leaves of kale, or a huge handful
- 1-2 cups of water
- 1 tablespoon flax seed

Strawberry BlackBerry Yogurt Coconut Green Smoothie

Ingredients

- 1 cup strawberries
- 1 cup blackberries
- 1 cup low-fat Greek yogurt
- 1 cup coconut water
- 1 cup spinach leaves
- 1 tablespoon chia seeds
- 1 cup ice

Coconut Avocado Cinnamon Banana Mint Green Smoothie

Ingredients

- juice of 1 fresh young coconut
- ½ small avocado
- 2 scoops of flesh from the coconut
- ½ tsp cinnamon
- ½ banana or ½ cup mixed berries (you can use frozen)
- 1 tablespoon chia seeds
- 1 teaspoon flaxseed oil
- 5 fresh mint leaves
- 2 large handfuls organic kale, stems trimmed
- 1 tablespoon powdered spirulina or your favorite green powder

Banana Mango Coconut Date Vanilla Green Smoothie

Ingredients

- 2 bananas
- 1 cup mango, chopped
- 1 cup young thai coconut water
- 3 pitted medjool dates
- ½ teaspoon vanilla bean powder
- 1 cup cucumber, chopped
- 3 celery stalks, chopped

Banana Vanilla Ginger Green Smoothie

Ingredients

- 2 bananas
- 2 teaspoons vanilla extract
- 1 inch ginger, finely shredded or pressed in garlic press
- 2 cups brewed chamomile tea
- 1 cup spinach

Pineapple Kiwi Cashew Green Smoothie

Ingredients

- 4 ounces pineapple
- 1 kiwi, peeled
- ½ teaspoon matcha powder
- ¼ cup raw cashews
- ½ ounces baby kale
- 1 cup water
- 1 cup ice

Orange Vanilla Carrot Smoothie

Ingredients

- 1 cup orange juice
- 1 orange, peeled and sliced into chunks
- ¾ cup vanilla almond milk
- 1 teaspoon vanilla extract
- 1 carrot, peeled and chopped
- 1 cup ice

Orange Blueberry Pineapple Smoothie

Ingredients

- ½ cup orange juice
- ¾ cup frozen blueberries
- ¾ cup frozen pineapple chunks
- 1 teaspoon chia seeds
- orange slices

Avocado Almond Date Green Smoothie

Ingredients

- ¼ ripe avocado
- ¾ cup unsweetened almond milk
- 1 teaspoon smooth unsalted almond butter
- 3 dates, pitted
- Handful of baby spinach
- 1 teaspoon vanilla extract
- 4 to 5 drops liquid stevia, to taste
- 2 ice cubes
- 1 teaspoon whole chia seeds, to serve
- 1 cup ice

Banana Strawberry Apple Green Smoothie

Ingredients

- 1 Banana
- 1 cup Strawberries
- 2 leaves Kale
- 1 Apple
- 1 tablespoon of ground Flax Seed
- ¼ cup of Walnuts
- 1 cup of your favorite liquid such as Oat Milk, Coconut Water, Rice Milk

Orange Blueberry Pineapple Coconut Smoothie

Ingredients

- ½ cup orange juice
- ¾ cup frozen blueberries
- ¾ cup frozen pineapple chunks
- 1 teaspoon chia seeds
- shredded coconut

Orange Blueberry Pineapple Pomegranate Smoothie

Ingredients

- ½ cup orange juice
- ¾ cup frozen blueberries
- ¾ cup frozen pineapple chunks
- 1 teaspoon chia seeds
- pomegranate seeds

Avocado Honey Smoothie

Ingredients

- 1 avocado, halved and pitted
- 1 cup low fat milk
- 1 tablespoon honey, plus more if needed
- 1 tablespoon chia seeds
- 4 whole ice cubes

Lemon Orange Green Smoothie

Ingredients

- 1 lemon
- 1 orange
- 1 cucumber
- 2 stalks celery (juiced)

Pear Banana Lime Pineapple Smoothie

Ingredients

- 1 cup pear
- ½ banana
- ¼ pineapple (juiced)
- ½ lime (fresh-squeezed juice)
- ½ cup almond milk or coconut milk
- 5 ice cubes

Apple Banana Almond Green Smoothie

Ingredients

- ½ apple
- 1 banana
- ½ cup spinach
- 2 celery stalks
- 1 tablespoon almond butter
- 5 ice cubes

Grape Pear Kiwi Mint Smoothie

Ingredients

- 1 cup grapes
- 1 pear
- 1-2 kiwi fruit, peeled
- 5 mint leaves
- 5 ice cubes

Chamomile Pineapple Pear Carrot Smoothie

Ingredients

- ½ cup of chamomile herbal tea
- ¼ cup pineapple
- 4 carrots (juiced)
- 1 cup of pear
- 3-4 drops of lavender tincture
- 5 ice cubes

Strawberry Yogurt Peach Smoothie

Ingredients

- 2½ cups strawberries
- ½ cup strawberry nectar
- 1 cup low-fat plain yogurt or strawberry yogurt
- 1 pitted peach
- 2 cups ground ice

Strawberry Yogurt Mango Smoothie

Ingredients

- 2½ cups strawberries
- ½ cup strawberry nectar
- 1 cup low-fat plain yogurt or strawberry yogurt
- 1 mango
- 2 cups ground ice

Strawberry Honey Smoothie

Ingredients

- 1 cup strawberries
- 1 tablespoon honey
- ¼ cup water
- 4 ice cubes

Avocado Banana Blueberry Yogurt Coconut Smoothie

Ingredients

- ½ avocado
- ½ banana
- ½ cup of blueberries,
- 1 tablespoon of coconut oil
- ¼ cup of plain, probiotic yogurt
- ¼ Tbsp. Himalayan pink salt
- 1 cup of raw milk
- water

Bonus 2 - Top "Stress Busting" Juices...

Raspberry Kiwi Watermelon Juice

Ingredients

- 1 cup of raspberries
- 2 kiwi fruit (no need to peel, just wash them)
- As much watermelon as you can easily drink

Papaya Strawberry Mint Juice

Ingredients

- ½ large papaya
- 1 cup of strawberries
- 1 handful of fresh mint, including the stalks

Apple Green Juice

Ingredients

- 2 green apples
- a bunch of spinach
- ½ a cucumber
- 1 stick celery
- ¼ lemon
- ½ inch ginger root (optional)

Carrot Green Juice

Ingredients

- 1 carrot
- 1 beetroot (medium)
- 2 radish
- 3 broccoli heads and stalks
- 1 stick of celery

Carrot Tomatoes Green Juice

Ingredients

- 1 carrot
- 2 medium tomatoes
- 1 small beetroot
- 2 celery sticks
- 3 to 4 parsley stems with leaves, roughly chopped
- 2 to 3 coriander (dhania) sprigs, roughly chopped
- 6 to 8 spinach (palak) leaves, roughly chopped
- crushed ice to serve

Apple Carrot Lemon Green Juice

Ingredients

- 2 apples
- 2 carrots
- ½ lemon
- 2 stalks of celery
- 1 cup of leafy greens (your choice)
- 2-4 sprigs of fresh lavender flowers per 1 cup of juice
- 4-6 sprigs per 1 cup of juice lemon balm

Carrot Apple Beet Green Juice

Ingredients

- 2 carrots
- ½ apple
- 1 large beet
- 1 cup parsley
- 1 inch. piece of ginger

Carrot Beet Green Juice

Ingredients

- 3 medium carrots.
- 2 stalks of celery.
- 1 large or 2 small beetsp
- an inch-long piece of ginger

Carrot Apple Green Juice

Ingredients

- 3 carrots, peeled
- 1 green apple, unpeeled
- 3 stalks of lemongrass
- 2 thumb-sized pieces fresh ginger root, unpeeled
- a pinch of sea salt

Blueberry Strawberry Beet Green Juice

Ingredients

- 1 cup blueberries
- ½ cup strawberries
- ½ medium beet
- 1 large leafy green
- 1½ cups milk or water

Apple Tomatoes Green Juice

Ingredients

- 2 apples
- 2 large tomatoes
- 1 large cucumber
- 2 branches of kale

Apple Pineapple Green Juice

Ingredients

- 2 apples
- ½ small pineapple
- 1 bunch of parsley
- ½ ahead of cabbage

Bonus 3 - Top "Stress Busting" Tips...

Stressful situations are not necessarily the problem. Some people will thrive on a particular circumstance; others will tolerate it, while still others will struggle with it. Slamming on your breaks to avoid a collision is a stress response, should last moments, and should be easy to shake off, and everybody is built to tolerate these bursts of stress hormones.

However, stress means different things to different people. Stress was an evolutionary advantage in ancient times, with a gene that triggers the "fight" or "flight" syndrome, but for the most part, it's obsolete in today's modern society, unless you happen to be a mom who had an auto accident and is trying to get to her kids, and even then, these bursts of stress hormones serve their purpose, but we are just not built to handle extended periods of stress.

Stress is meant to be a short term response, but in modern society, people often experience periods of chronic stress, leading to a wide range of symptoms. Part of the problem is your body quickly breaks down proteins for the energy needed for fight or flight, so anyone who is chronically stressed needs to replenish these proteins frequently.

Chronic stress will inhibit the immune response, cardiovascular function, neuroendocrine function and central nervous system function, which can manifest itself in many ways for different people.

Medical studies have shown that the physical signs of stress contributes to overeating, belly fat, high blood pressure, headaches, migraines, stomachaches, diarrhea, constipation, insomnia, fatigue, irritability, restlessness, burnout, worry, tension, faintness, tingling, impatience, shaking, nail biting, fear, sweating, panic attacks, confusion, obsessive and intrusive thoughts, memory and concentration problems, anxious, anxiety, depression, strokes, heart disease, diabetes, colitis, asthma, rheumatism, skin allergies, sexual difficulties, hardening of the arteries, ulcers, breathing problems, kidney disorders, and weakening of the immune system, which can lead to a host of infections, chronic conditions and despises.

Chronic stress is a serious condition and both directly and indirectly kills people. Stress is the polar opposite of relaxation, which is the state your body needs to rejuvenate and effectively fight disease. Stress suppresses many body functions that are not necessary for fight or flight, so things like the healing process just don't happen, with the exception of blood clotting for a wound.

Severe stress for any extended period of time can be physiologically and physiologically debilitating and can take a severe emotional toil with otherwise healthy individuals, so getting a handle on stress is the single best thing anyone can do for themselves, especially when fighting a disease.

Stress is the real underlying enemy for anyone who is coping with related symptoms, struggling with mental and physical health related conditions, allowing stress to affect everyday activities, trying to bounce-back from any disease and needs a well-functioning immune system, struggling with low energy, fatigue or burnout, or is just having difficulty maintaining their livelihood because of stress or related symptoms, or getting sick too frequently.

Fortunately, severe stress, often referred to as anxiety or depression, can be treatable with holistic approaches, nutrition, exercise, sleep, along with any combination of approaches covered in this book.

The great news is stress improvements can often be immediate, but will likely take some on-going effort to build up a strong tolerance and resilience, resulting in substantial improvements to overall health and wellbeing. It is all much easier and enjoyable than you might expect too, making stress manageable in a way that suites your lifestyle, instead of letting stress manage you, or even run you over.

Anything you can do to improve your overall health, and get a handle on stress, is also great for your immune system, making it harder to get sick, having more days where you feel on top of your game, and solving the underlying problem contributing to any challenge or condition you might be struggling with.

Physical activity, a healthy diet, and a good night's rest are all helpful at reducing stress. Try getting as much as 8-9 hours of uninterrupted sleep as night. If insomnia is part of the problem, you can try some natural remedies that include Melatonin or herbs that act as sedatives.

Although laughter may not be the easiest thing to do when you are stressed, it is one of the best medicines for stress symptoms. It reduces stress hormone levels, releases tension and brings positive physiological changes, so hit a comic club, watch your favorite sitcom, do a prank, or do whatever gets a laugh out of you.

Breathing exercises are immediately beneficial. Simply take a deep breath from your diaphragm, slowly through your noise, while your belly expands, exhale slowly and repeat a few times. Slow deep breathing with long deep breathes serves to relax the nerves system.

Heating up the body with a warm bath, sun bathing, warm fire, sauna, steam room, or even a hot cup of tea, will reduce muscle tension and anxiety and makes you more relaxed and improves mood, including serotonin release.

Listening to music can be a great way to relax and help with stress, has a calming effect while facing the day's stressors, but choose music that already resonates with you, that you already know will lift your spirits and help you get back into the groove.

Take a forest bath, known as Skinrin-yoku by the Japanese, which more accurately translates to a short walk in the woods with all the outdoor odors and background sounds of streams, proven to reduce stress hormone levels and make you more relaxed in no time.

Relieve tension and stress by applying pressure to your pressure points. Simply breathe deeply and apply steady pressure for a few minutes. Common pressure points to do include the temples, the point between both eyebrows, the back of the neck slightly below the scull, about an inch down from your shoulders, towards the back of your neck, or anywhere you feel aching when you apply pressure.

Mantras are an excellent way to silence the self-critical voice that can result with stress. Try coming up with a manta of the day, or just as needed, as part of your routine mental exercise. Simple mantras might go something like "I'm Ready for This" or "Bring it". Repeat your manta of the day at least several times, with several successions. The Ahh meditation technique or even staring at a burning candle serves to relax the mind, allow focus, and reduce stress symptoms.

Enjoy aromatherapy for stress relief, to become more energized, relaxed and present. Lavender is associated with feelings of contentment, cognitive performance, and mood. Peppermint is particularly good for stress, memory and alertness and is a great pick-me-up. Vanilla Extract is often readily available and is very uplifting for your mood. Basil, hay, eucalyptus, rose, and thyme oils are also very soothing.

You can do acupuncture too, it has been proven to reduce stress hormone levels. I've never tried it personally, but my sister swears by it and some insurance companies will pay for it.

Massage therapy feels great and is a very popular way to relax and relieve stress, preferably a full body massage.

Get yourself a great life coach who is really in the now like Kidest OM. If anyone can get you out of a funk, she can, and then some; she is very inspirational.

Kidest OM on YouTube
https://www.youtube.com/results?search_query=Kidest+OM

Do something you enjoy, like a hobby, crafts, art, dancing, volunteer work, etc. Enjoy a good game with friends or play something relaxing to take your mind off of stressors.

Gardening can be a great stress reliever. It combines satisfaction for your creation with exercise and getting outside in the sun and enjoying the scenery.

Do something active like a sport, including racket ball, swimming, basketball, volleyball, skiing, or just take a long walk, etc. These can all be fantastic stress relievers that get you in a different frame of mind and work in minutes.

Playing with and caring for pets are a great way to help you focus on the moment.

Roll with the punches and when you get the opportunity to be proactive, take it. Don't let yourself become a victim or feel helpless, that's the true path to the dark side, stress.

Did you know that loneliness and social isolation are twice as dangerous as obesity for mortality? Make a point to get together with family and friends. A lifestyle that allows you to feel safe, secure, empowered or important makes you more resilient to stress.

Accept that there are circumstances beyond your control, so there is no point aimlessly dwelling on them.

Maintain a positive attitude and outlook, don't let yourself be pessimistic.

Takes 15 minute breaks when you feel overwhelmed, to relax and reflect. Learn relaxation techniques like meditation, yoga and breathing.

These Bonus "Stress Busting" Healthy Tips are complements and excerpts from Healthy Vibrations, Discover Your Highly Vibrant Wellbeing, an excellent self-help book to further heighten your awareness about your stress, your health, your energy levels, raising your vibrations, and restoring inner peace, joy, and happiness, while helping you become more successful than ever and activate your mind body for awakenings of all kinds.

Discover how to energize your life effectively with nutrition, sound and music therapy, more effective stress management techniques, and mind body techniques.

Apply these amazing techniques for prevention and wellbeing, or for chronic conditions and disease, including anxiety, depression and fatigue.

Raise your vibrations to new heights to expand your consciousness, creativity, intuition and awareness, become healthier, more energetic, and increase your attraction like a magnet in a "like" attracts "like" kind of way.

Learn to enjoy life more with this incredible journey, greater personal power, clarity of mind, inner peace, love and joy, as your life flows with synchronicity, with greater intuition and awareness, you effortlessly manifest your personal desires reflected in your external life. This is a great place to be and what should be a major layover on any path to enlightenment, while exploring and gaining experience.

There are so many benefits to living a healthier, highly vibrational life and the techniques illustrated throughout this book can be adopted in part, at your own pace, and on your own terms, so you can begin to work up some momentum starting right away.

Although this book is loaded with informational and inspirational resources and links throughout, the final chapter covers advanced tools for your tool belt, including advanced meditation techniques and loads of free, effective and healthy music downloads for your mix. Most of these techniques are absolutely free to get started with right away.

This book will help you take everything to the next level with progressively increasing health, wellbeing, vibrations, awakenings, and even the opportunity to experience the ultimate reality for yourself, in a highly vibrant and joyful way!

Get **Healthy Vibrations, Discover Your Highly Vibrant Wellbeing** at Amazon in Paperback, Kindle, or Any Device App Edition while promotional prices last. Healthy Vibrations is available to Kindle Unlimited Customers free of charge.

https://www.amazon.com/dp/1530003458

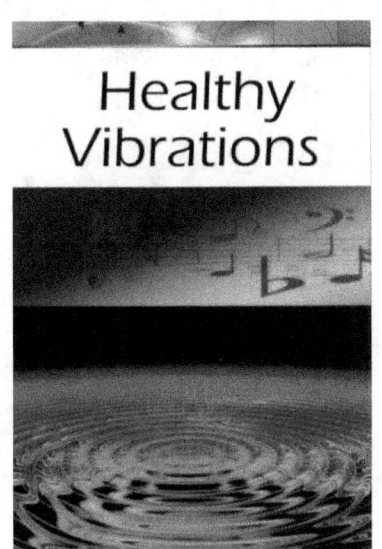 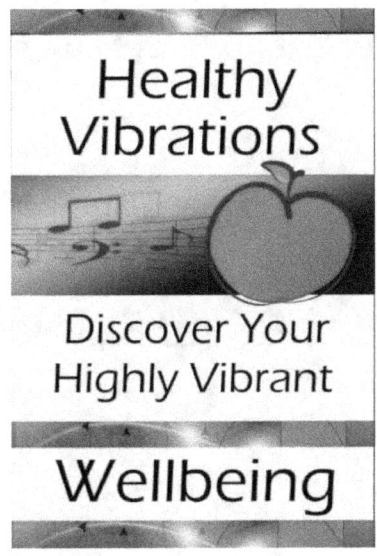

Bonus 5 - If you need **Top 50 Best "Stress Busting" Smoothies** in any other formats, for any other devices you have, or if you have made a purchase and want it for immediate family or close friends, you can get it at Smashswords in the formats (ePub, Mobi, PDF, LRF, PDB, HTML, Text)

Use Coupon Code BX62S

https://www.smashwords.com/books/view/618259